Reflux and Oesophageal Problems
Second Edition

T0231167

Reflux and Oesophageal Problems

Second Edition

John R Bennett, MD, FRCP
Honorary Clinical Professor of Medicine
and Consultant Physician

University of Hull

Hull Royal Infirmary,

Hull, UK

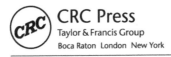

CRC Press
Taylor & Francis Group
Boca Raton London New York

CRC Press is an imprint of the
Taylor & Francis Group, an **informa** business

CRC Press
Taylor & Francis Group
6000 Broken Sound Parkway NW, Suite 300
Boca Raton, FL 33487-2742

Contents

Compared with the complexity of secretory and motor functions of the rest of the gut, the oesophagus is a relatively simple tube, acting as a conduit for food and fluid to enter the gut, or occasionally for undesired contents to be ejected. Nevertheless, the oesphagus is an actively motile organ with two important sphincters at its ends. It is also quite prone to disease. To some extent this may be the consequence of modern life: smoking, alcohol, obesity and perhaps other environmental toxins are partly responsible.

This pocketbook deals with the main symptoms of oesophageal disorders, and discusses the management of some of them.

Heartburn and Related Disorders

Background
Major clinical causes
Symptoms and diagnosis
Tests
Management
An approach to treatment
Complications of gastro-oesophageal reflux

Background

Heartburn is a common symptom that is often self-treated. Recent surveys, for example, show that two-thirds of the population sometimes have heartburn, though only about one-third of these consult their doctor about it. The cause is frequently gastro-oesophageal reflux, but other alimentary disorders may also lead to it. For instance:

- Hiatus hernia
- Flatulent dyspepsia
- Peptic ulceration
- Carcinoma of the pylorus
- Carcinoma of the cardia

Conversely, gastro-oesophageal reflux may cause pains of quite a different nature from heartburn, and these are discussed on pages 14 and 16.

There is a danger that heartburn may be dismissed as trivial, either by the patient or the practitioner. Yet many people suffer much discomfort from it. Heartburn can also restrict activity. If inadequately treated there may be a greater likelihood of complications (e.g. stricture or haemorrhage) and if the best form of medical therapy is not devised, the patient may finish up by having unnecessary surgery (see page 32).

Chest pains

The oesophagus may give rise to pain other than heartburn, probably by motor changes ('spasm'). This pain may be of any character, but is often described as 'gripping' or 'knife-like'. The pains are usually central sternal in origin, but may radiate widely to the abdomen, back, neck and arms. They are sometimes very severe. The character, radiation and severity of the pain may cause diagnostic difficulty, readily simulating cardiac, biliary or duodenal pain (see pages 14 and 16).

The major clinical causes of heartburn are:

- Gastro-oesophageal reflux
- Reflux oesophagitis
- Hiatus hernia
- Flatulent dyspepsia

Gastro-oesophageal reflux

Modern techniques of continuously measuring oesophageal acidity show that everyone squirts small amounts of gastric contents into their oesophagus several times a day. When this becomes abnormally frequent, or large in amount-because of incompetence of the normal barrier mechanisms at the gastro-oesophageal junction-it is referred to as gastro-oesophageal reflux, which leads to reflux oesophagitis.

Reflux oesophagitis

This is inflammation of the lower oesophageal mucosa caused by gastro-oesophageal reflux. It can be diagnosed endoscopi-cally (Figure 1), when lines of inflamed or ulcerated mucosa are seen extending up the oesophagus, or microscopically in biopsies taken at the time of endoscopy.

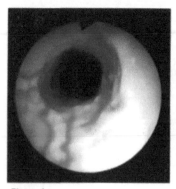

Figure 1
Endoscopic view of oesophagitis.
(Courtesy of Professor G Tytgat.)

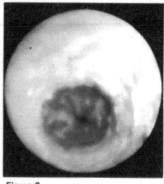

Figure 2
The characteristic white exudate in
monilial oesophagitis.

Oesophagitis can less frequently be caused by other sorts of damage, including infections (especially moniliasis, Figure 2) and swallowed corrosives (Figure 3), including drugs such as non-steroidal anti-inflammatory drugs (NSAIDs), tetracycline, potassium chloride and others (see page 46).

Hiatus hernia

Patients with gastro-oesophageal reflux often have a sliding hiatus hernia, in which the gastro-oesophageal junction and a segment of stomach herniate through the diaphragm from the abdomen into the thorax. However, a sliding hiatus hernia does not always produce reflux, and may be symptomless. Recent research suggests that a more important effect of a hiatus hernia may be in delaying oesophageal emptying to allow refluxed juices to 'yo-yo' up and down. Whether a barium meal (Figure 4) shows a hiatus hernia or not will depend on the enthusiasm of the radiologist. It is a pity that, for historical reasons, reflux symptoms are frequently labelled as being 'due to hiatus hernia'. Patients are often unduly worried about this label, fearing well-known complications characteristic of inguinal hernias (e.g. strangulation, incarceration, etc), and unreasonably assuming that they are likely to need surgical treatment.

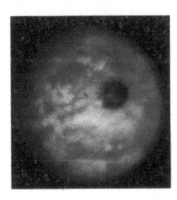

Figure 3
Endoscopic view of oesophagitis
caused by swallowed corrosive.

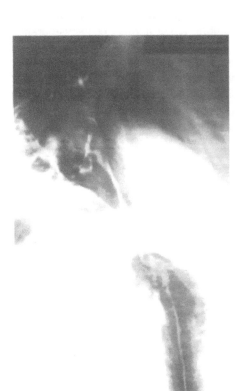

Figure 4
Barium meal showing
hiatus hernia.

Flatulent dyspepsia

This embraces a number of symptoms, including upper abdominal fullness, nausea, easy satiety, anorexia, morning vomiting, belching and heartburn. Although this condition is not fully understood, it may be due predominantly to disordered antral and duodenal motility with duodeno-gastric reflux. Alcohol abuse, excessive smoking and poor dietetics may cause similar symptoms, and anxiety can be a factor. While heartburn may partly respond to appropriate anti-reflux measures, other symptoms such as distension, satiety, nausea and belching will not. Motility-enhancing drugs may help with these.

Flatulent dyspepsia occurs in many patients with gallstones, though an equal number have normal cholecystograms. Removal of the gall bladder cures these symptoms in fewer than half of these patients. There is therefore little purpose in a 'routine' search for gall bladder disease in patients with reflux symptoms, though if a patient with gallstones has significant reflux oesophagitis, consideration may be given to performing an anti-reflux procedure at the same time as a cholecystectomy.

The symptoms set out below are indicative of gastro-oesophageal reflux, but some symptoms warn of possible alternative diagnoses and certainly indicate a need for further investigation by endoscopy (Figure 5).

Heartburn

An accurate diagnosis of heartburn is important, though this does not necessarily mean a lot of tests, and may be based mainly on the patient's history. (For details of tests available for diagnosis, see pages 18–22.) However, always beware of the heartburn which signals some other disease process (e.g. duo-denal ulcer, gastric ulcer, or carcinoma at the pylorus or in the gastric fundus). Points ('alarm symptoms') that should lead to early investigation are:

- Weight loss
- Dysphagia
- Vomiting
- Lack of response to medical treatment

Heartburn is the commonest symptom of gastro-oesophageal reflux, and is due to irritation of the oesophageal mucosa by refluxed juice. The discomfort or pain is usually burning in char-

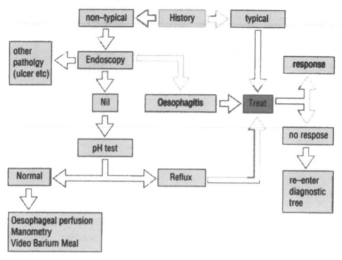

Figure 5
Diagnosis of gastro–oesophageal reflux.

acter and felt behind the sternum, often seeming to rise from the epigastrium towards or into the throat. It may radiate into the back. Such heartburn occurs intermittently, particularly 30 minutes after meals, or on exercise (especially if any bending is involved). It can also occur after lying down and may even waken patients from sleep. A large meal, particularly one with an excess of fat or alcohol, is especially prone to cause heartburn. However, this discomfort often disappears quickly on drinking water or milk, or after taking an antacid.

Odynophagia

This is a diagnostic symptom of oesophagitis (reflux, infective or corrosive) where the patient experiences a burning discomfort when swallowing hot or alcoholic drinks.

Regurgitation
The entry of acid or bitter (bile) fluid into the mouth is an obvious indication of gastro-oesophageal reflux.

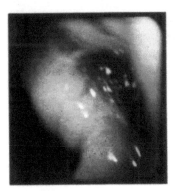

Figure 6
Endoscopic view of bleeding ulcer within a hiatus hernia.

Bleeding

Overt haemorrhage from reflux oesophagitis accounts for about 4 per cent of all cases of gastrointestinal haemorrhage. Occult bleeding is also uncommon.

Gastrointestinal endoscopy is the only way to identify the site of a haemorrhage. Hiatus hernia, diagnosed radiologically, cannot be regarded as an adequate explanation because the hernia itself does not bleed; haemorrhage arises from a related cause such as severe oesophagitis, or a mucosal tear. In cases of occult bleeding or iron deficiency, endoscopic confirmation of a site of bleeding is essential. If no abnormality is seen, the lower gastrointestinal tract may need investigation.

Oesophageal ulcers, or gastric ulcers in the intrathoracic portion of a herniated stomach, bleed more often than uncomplicated oesophagitis (Figure 6).

Respiratory problems

Some patients with chronic bronchitis, recurrent pneumonia, or asthma, have gastro-oesophageal reflux. However, it is always difficult to be sure if reflux is the cause of respiratory problems. Sometimes the conditions are coincidental and at times the intrathoracic pressure changes caused by respiratory problems may predispose to gastro-oesophageal reflux. Nevertheless, reflux is worth considering in any patient with a recurrent pulmonary problem where there is no other likely causative factor. (Tests for determining reflux oesophagitis are outlined on pages 18–22.)

If there is a free reflux, the patient may benefit from anti-reflux surgery, though at present no pre-operative test offers a satisfactory prediction of outcome. By the same token, patients with reflux symptoms who have asthma or bronchitis should always be carefully investigated as they might well benefit from anti-reflux surgery.

Chest pains

Consciousness of the fact that chest pain may be a harbinger of sudden death may tend to concentrate the minds of patients and doctors on the heart. Yet, in about a fifth of all patients admitted to hospital with chest pains, the cause is in the oesophagus.

- From the oesophageal standpoint, the investigations may include perfusion of the oesophagus with acid to precipitate pain (which the patient may recognize), endoscopy to show oesophagitis, measurement of acid reflux using intraluminal pH monitoring, or manometric measurements of oesophageal motility to detect 'spasm'.

- From a cardiac standpoint, investigations will include exercise electrocardiograms, thallium perfusion scans and coronary arteriograms may be necessary to rule out or to demonstrate coronary artery disease.

The difficulty of differentiating cardiac and oesophageal pains is compounded because pain from the gullet may be brought on by exertion or emotion, just as in angina pectoris. Detailed investigations of the heart and oesophagus may be needed before any certainty of the cause can be established.

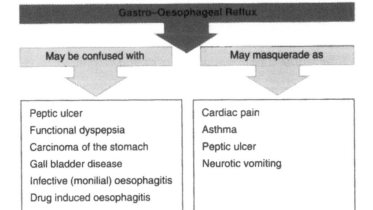

Gastro–Oesophageal Reflux	
May be confused with	May masquerade as
Peptic ulcer Functional dyspepsia Carcinoma of the stomach Gall bladder disease Infective (monilial) oesophagitis Drug induced oesophagitis	Cardiac pain Asthma Peptic ulcer Neurotic vomiting

Table 1
Differential diagnosis.

Marked epigastric discomfort
Although the discomfort of reflux oesophagitis may be predominantly felt in the epigastrium, marked epigastric pain must raise the question of peptic ulceration. Ulcers in the stomach or duodenum-especially those close to the pylorus-may cause reflux by interfering with gastric emptying. Periodicity of symptoms (with weeks or months of freedom) also hints at a possible duodenal ulcer.

Dysphagia
The condition is discussed more fully on page 40. A sensation of hold-up at the lower end of the sternum as food is swallowed may occur in reflux oesophagitis, but if it is more than mild and occasional, it suggests some additional problem such as stricture, an associated motility disorder, or a carcinoma. Indeed, carcinoma of the lower oesophagus or gastric fundus may masquerade as 'simple' gastro-oesophageal reflux by infiltrating the cardia, rendering it rigid and incompetent and thus allowing reflux to occur.

Endoscopy should be done in any patient whose heartburn does not readily respond to treatment.

Differential diagnosis of reflux oesophagitis

Peptic Ulcer

Gastro-oesophageal reflux often complicates or coexists with peptic ulceration, probably because of changes in gastric motility and the acid and bile content of the gastric juice. In a patient with reflux symptoms, an ulcer may be suggested by unusually rapid progress of the symptoms (e.g. epigastric pain as well as heartburn), or periodicity of the duodenal type. A peptic ulcer should be looked for radiologically or endoscopically in most patients with reflux symptoms.

Cardiac pain

Typical oesophageal pain is readily differentiated from typical cardiac pain and the main characteristics are given in Table 2. However pain is frequently not typical. Oesophageal pain may be gripping; cardiac pain may be burning. Oesophageal pain may come after exercise or emotion; cardiac pain may seem to be caused by meals. Relief by antacids or nitrates can be misleading because of placebo response. Moreover, because both are common conditions both types of pain may occur in the same patients (Figure 7). Detailed investigation of the heart and the oesophagus may be needed before any certainty of the cause can be established. Careful elicitation of all details of the pain should lead to an accurate diagnosis in most cases, but electrocardiograms (perhaps after exercise) and tests for reflux oesophagitis may be needed. Provocative tests for oesophageal pain (e.g. acid perfusion, drugs like edrophonium, or balloon distension) can be employed.

Typical pain	
Cardiac	**Oesophageal**
Central, or across chest	Substernal
Uncommon in the back	Quite often radiates to back
Often radiates to throat, arms, even hands	May radiate to upper arms, rarely beyond
Tight; gripping	Burning; soreness
On exertion	After meals
Relieved by nitrates or rest	Relieved by antacids
Associated Symptoms	**Associated Symptoms**
Dyspnoea	Odynophagia
	Dysphagia
	Belch
	Hiccup

Table 2
Characteristics of oesophageal and cardiac pain

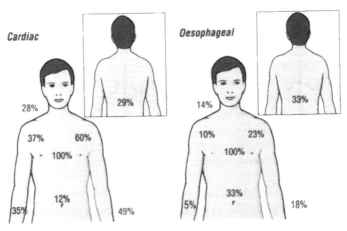

Figure 7
Frequency of radiation to various anatomical sites of cardiac and oesophageal pain.

In the diagnosis of gastro-oesophageal reflux, there are two purposes:

(1) To demonstrate that the patient's symptoms are due to reflux and not to any other disease (e.g. cardiac, biliary, etc)

(2) To show whether the reflux is 'primary', or associated with upper alimentary pathology.

All tests have their limitations and this should always be borne in mind, however persuasive the report may sound.

In many patients the diagnosis of reflux oesophagitis is easy. The patient complains of heartburn with the characteristic postural and dietary associations, without dysphagia, vomiting or weight loss. In these individuals, tests are unnecessary and the treatment outlined on pages 31–32 can be given. However, follow-up is desirable to ensure that the therapy has given relief and that no new symptoms have arisen.

Some patients do not improve with a simple regimen and there the diagnosis will need to be reconsidered and a barium meal or endoscopy performed to ensure there is no other disease apparent. If uncomplicated reflux oesophagitis still appears to be the problem, a firmer enforcement of dietary and tobacco restrictions and adherence to medication may be needed. Additionally, the patient should be asked to elevate the head of his bed (on bricks or blocks, for instance) approximately 10 cm to reduce nocturnal reflux and improve oesophageal emptying.

If three or four weeks of the above treatment bring no improvement, a consultant's opinion should be sought. Endoscopic examination will be needed and, possibly, functional studies of the oesophagus and stomach. However, the great majority of patients do improve, especially if they adhere to the advice.

An upper gastrointestinal endoscopy is necessary in the following instances, not only to confirm reflux oesophagitis but particularly to discover a peptic ulcer or carcinoma of the cardia or pylorus which may cause reflux symptoms:

- If the symptoms are unexpected and are less than typical
- If the symptoms are associated with epigastric pain or dysphagia
- If the symptoms fail to respond to treatment.

Equally, if the chest pain is not typically oesophageal, and especially if it resembles cardiac pain, then a more careful assessment is required-particularly using tests to provoke oesophageal pain and to measure reflux quantitatively.

Barium swallow and meal

This test is relatively simple and quite comfortable for the patient. It will reveal most peptic ulcers or carcinomas. It may also demonstrate oesophageal anatomy and show a hiatus hernia-although a hiatus hernia does not in itself mean that there is gastro-oesophageal reflux, or that reflux is the cause of a patient's symptoms (see Figure 3). Reflux of barium may be seen, but it is an insensitive test dependent upon the radiologist's technique and cannot be relied on.

Barium radiology will not usually show any oesophageal abnormality due to oesophagitis unless there is an ulcer or a stricture. Its value is mainly to rule out alternative or causative pathology.

Upper gastrointestinal endoscopy

Although a little more uncomfortable and slightly more hazardous to the patient than a barium X-ray, endoscopy is more informative in patients with oesophageal symptoms. It will detect peptic ulcers and carcinomas, as well as permitting mucosal biopsies. It enables a visual assessment of oesophagitis (see Figure 1), although in up to 50 per cent of patients with undoubted gastro-oesophageal reflux no abnormality is seen.

Oesophageal perfusion

If there is any doubt as to the origin of the symptoms, the best test to perform is probably oesophageal perfusion - sometimes known as the Bernstein test. If a drip of 0.1 N hydrochloric acid is introduced into the oesophagus through an indwelling tube and it accurately reproduces the patient's discomfort or pain within 10 to 20 minutes, and a control perfusion does not, then it is likely that the diagnosis is gastro-oesophageal reflux.

Intraluminal pH measurements

Although acid is not the sole cause of reflux oesophagitis, acid does reflux abnormally in the great majority of patients with this disorder. Thus, using a small glass pH electrode (Figure 8) to measure the frequency with which acid spurts into the lower oesophagus is a relatively simple method of quantifying reflux. It is now best to monitor oesophageal pH for 24 hours, using a mobile recorder. Various measurements (e.g. the frequency of acid spurts, their average duration, or the proportion of recording time under pH4 or pH5) may be measured and compared with results obtained in normal subjects. Of course, everyone has a few episodes of acid reflux every day, but in patients with reflux oesophagitis their frequency and duration are increased (Figure 9).

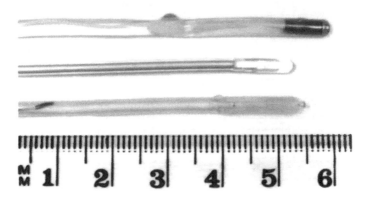

Figure 8
(a) Combined glass reference pH electrode (Inglold);
(b) antimony pH electrode;
(c) combined antimony and reference pH electrode.

Oesophageal scintiscanning

If an isotope-labelled substance such as ^{99m}Tc sulphur colloid is instilled into the stomach, it can be detected by a gamma-camera. If some standard provocation is used (e.g. abdominal binder, or provocative manoeuvres), reflux of the isotope can be detected and quantified. In accuracy, this sensitive test is comparable to pH monitoring but requires a gamma-camera. Besides the patient sometimes finds the abdominal binder uncomfortable at high pressures.

Oesophageal manometry

Pressure recording in the oesophagus makes it possible to measure lower oesophageal sphincter tone or 'squeeze', and to assess oesophageal peristalsis. This test is not very helpful in the diagnosis of gastro-oesophageal reflux because although gastro-oesophageal sphincter tone tends to be lower in reflux subjects, there is a considerable overlap with the normal population (Figure 10).

Manometry is often used in patients who have responded poorly to treatment, or as a preliminary to surgery to ensure that oesophageal peristalsis is normal. It will detect peristaltic failure (e.g. in systemic sclerosis in which reflux oesophagitis is common), or motor abnormalities (e.g. diffuse oesophageal spasm) which may themselves cause oesophageal pain in the absence of gastro-oesophageal reflux. Manometry is also being used increasingly in those patients whose chest pain was at first thought to be of a cardiac origin. Many of these patients have abnormal oesophageal spasm as the cause of pain (Figure 11).

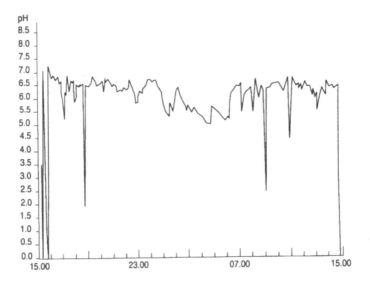

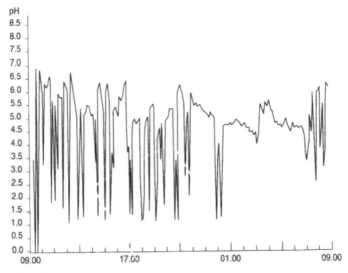

Figure 9
Recordings of lower oesophageal pH over 24 hours.
(a) Normal person (pH<4.0 0.8%).
(b) Patient with moderate gastro-oesophageal reflux (pH<4.0 8.7% total; 10.2% ambulant; 6.6% recumbent).

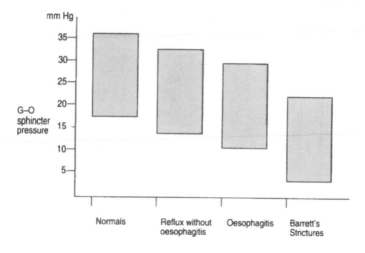

Figure 10
Range of gastro–oesophageal sphincter pressures in normals and patients with reflux of different severities.

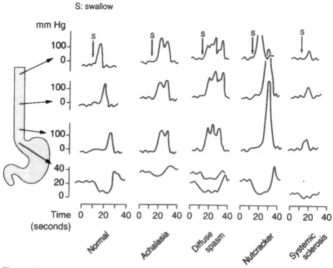

Figure 11
Manometric changes in some motility disorders.

The oesophagitis spiral

It is not understood why some patients develop gastro-oesophageal reflux, and the causative factors set out below vary in importance from patient to patient. There must be an initial failure of the gastro-oesophageal barrier, sometimes for anatomical reasons, but usually because of disordered neuromuscular function leading to frequent 'inappropriate' relaxation of the sphincter with accompanying acid reflux.

Ultimately, in every patient, worsening oesophagitis generates increasing functional failure - the sphincter weakens, clearing declines, and mucosal sensitivity increases. This has been termed the 'vicious spiral' whose direction needs reversing if the problem is to be cured. Except in trivial cases where a few doses of any antacid are enough to give relief, attention must be paid to each contributing component (Figure 12).

Causative factors
These abnormalities can be classified as :

- The reflux barrier
- Gastric factors
- The refluxed juice
- Oesophageal emptying
- Mucosal sensitivity

The reflux barrier

Irritant juices enter the oesophagus because the normal barrier to reflux at the cardia is weakened. Susceptible individuals may have some anatomical abnormality that alters the relative disposition of the structures around the oesophageal hiatus, which constitute the barrier to reflux. The gastro-oesophageal sphincter (anatomically invisible, but detectable by pressure measurements, see page 21) either may be permanently weak, or may respond inadequately to stressful forces, or may relax at inappropriate moments. None of these failings is readily corrected, but factors known to weaken the sphincter should be avoided, and agents which strengthen the sphincter can be employed. Oesophagitis may itself reduce sphincter tone. However, this vicious circle may be reversed by treating the disease since the sphincter tone may then improve as the inflammation diminishes. Equally, sphincter tone may be diminished by the following factors, which are best avoided by the heartburn suffer:

- Large meals, probably due to stretching of the gastric fundus
- Fatty meals, probably induced by the effects of the hormone cholecystokinin
- Smoking, coffee, or eating chocolate or spices – by their pharmacological effect
- Pregnancy and the contraceptive pill – by their hormonal effect.

Improvement of the barrier mechanism is obtained by the use of drugs or alginate preparations.

- Drugs: metoclopramide, domperidone, cholinergics (e.g. bethanechol) and cisapride all elevate gastro-oesophageal sphincter pressure, cisapride having the most consistent and longest-lasting effect.
- Alginate preparations: alginates form a glutinous raft floating on the gastric contents, which by its physical properties reduces acid reflux. Antacid contained in the preparation also neutralizes any refluxing acid (Figure 13).

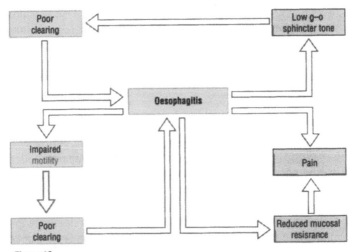

Figure 12
Oesophagitis spiral.

Gastric factors

If the volume of gastric contents is great, then reflux is likely to be increased. If gastric emptying is slow (as it is in perhaps half the patients with reflux oesophagitis), then more reflux will occur. The intragastric volume should be kept small by the patient avoiding large meals and fizzy drinks. In addition, gastric emptying can be speeded up, and the volume in the stomach reduced, by the avoidance of fatty meals and the use of a prokinetic drug such as metoclopramide or cisapride. Reflux oesophagitis is worse in the obese but improves with slimming, though it is uncertain why this is so.

The refluxed juice

Acid and pepsin are the chief constituents which cause and perpetuate heartburn. Occasionally, bile, trypsin and other constituents of duodenal juice may play a part, but this is unusual with an intact stomach. Gastric acid is the main producer of pain in almost all heartburn sufferers, and it is one of the causative factors of the oesophagitis. Some reflux patients secrete more 'basal' acid than normal. It can be neutralized by any antacid taken frequently (say, every hour). This explains the popularity of antacids as heartburn relievers, and they remain the most common and convenient remedy. When antacids are combined with an alginate preparation, the combination has acid-neutralizing qualities added to the mechanical 'stopper' effect.

Inhibition of acid secretion will obviously diminish the volume and concentration of the acid available for reflux. Anti-secretory drugs (H_2-antagonists and proton pump inhibitors) reduce gastric secretion, diminishing the volume of gastric contents and the concentration of acid available for reflux. The dose of an H_2-antagonist may be titrated upwards to optimum effect; proton pump inhibitors are more powerful. Pepsin damages the mucosa, but only in an acid medium (hence the term 'peptic oesophagitis'), but so far there are no effective anti-pepsins available for use. However, raising the pH by antacids or suppression of acid secretion will considerably inhibit peptic activity. The place of bile in causing oesophagitis is still uncertain, but it might theoretically play a part by enabling acid-peptic juices to penetrate the mucosa. Some antacids have weak bile-binding properties, but stronger agents (e.g. cholestyramine) are unpleasant to take and, in any case, leave the stomach and oesophagus too quickly to work effectively. When reflux of duodenal juices seems to be a major factor (e.g. after gastroenterostomy) a surgical procedure ('Roux-en-Y') to divert them can be used if oesophagitis is severe, especially if complicated by the development of a benign stricture.

Oesophageal emptying
The normal function of the oesophagus is to propel its contents into the stomach by peristalsis. This applies to swallowed as well as refluxed material. Emptying of a paralysed oesophagus (e.g. in scleroderma) will obviously be poor. However, peristalsis often becomes ineffective or even absent as oesophagitis increases; consequently, refluxed juices remain longer in contact with the mucosa. If oesophagitis is to be improved, the oesophagus must be kept empty of irritants, not only by pre-

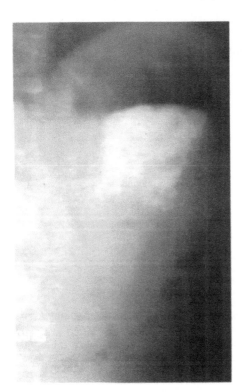

Figure 13
X–ray showing alginate raft (opacified with barium) floating on gastric contents.

vention of reflux but also by encouragement of emptying. Gravity helps, so the patient should avoid bending; having the bedhead raised will assist the process. Frequent swallowing (induced by sucking antacid tablets, for instance) stimulates primary peristaltic contractions, and the alkaline saliva itself helps to neutralize acid. Cisapride strengthens the cleansing peristaltic waves. As oesophagitis heals, the abnormally delayed clearing tends to improve. Thus, in the long term, the best course is to cure the oesophagitis.

Mucosal sensitivity
The susceptibility of the oesophageal mucosa varies from person to person, certainly with regard to pain sensitivity, and some mucosae may resist peptic digestion better than others.

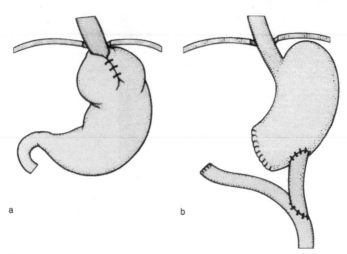

Figure 14
Some operations for control of reflux: (a) Nissen and (b) Roux–en–Y.

Cigarette smoke, alcohol and some drugs (especially aspirin and other NSAIDs) decrease mucosal resistance and allow easier penetration of damaging H^+ ions into the mucosa. We are relatively ignorant about ways of improving mucosal resistance, apart from avoiding obvious irritants such as spices, citrus juices, smoking and alcohol, and drugs such as NSAIDs. As oesophagitis heals the mucosa becomes less sensitive.

An approach to treatment

Medical treatment

The first measures to adopt are those which are simple and inexpensive yet, if followed, are extremely effective-often more valuable than any drug.

- The obese must be slimmed
- Smokers must abandon cigarettes, cigars, etc
- Intake of fat, coffee, chocolate and spices should be reduced
- Drugs likely to worsen oesophagitis (e.g. corticosteroids, NSAIDs, potassium chloride) should, if possible, be stopped or certainly be reduced in dose.

A simple antacid (preferably in tablet form to encourage salivation and swallowing) should be taken frequently (every hour or two) whether there are symptoms or not. An antacid-alginate combination can be prescribed, to be taken after meals and at bedtime. If response to this is incomplete an H_2-antagonist should be prescribed, and may need to be titrated to a high dose (e.g. ranitidine 300 mg twice daily, famotidine 40 mg twice daily). For greater acid suppression a proton pump should be used (e.g. lanzoprazole 30 mg, omeprazole 20 mg, best given with a meal).

If symptoms are inadequately controlled after a month of this, the patient should elevate the bedhead by 10 cm, and cisapride can be added, particularly if there is noticeable regurgitation.

Once symptoms are controlled, that level of therapy should be maintained for about three months in the hope of healing oesophagitis and perhaps allowing restoration of normal oesophageal function. Some clinicians verify oesophagitis healing by repeat endoscopy but this is not obligatory.

Medication may then gradually be reduced to whatever level is sufficient to control symptoms. This means that some patients will require 'maintenance medication', but others may stop drugs entirely, possibly needing repeat courses from time to time.

Surgery

Operative treatment for uncomplicated reflux is never the first choice as all anti-reflux operations have a success rate of under 80 per cent. They not only carry the risks and problems of all major surgery, but often prove unnecessary once proper medical treatment has been established. In addition, a radiologist's report of a sliding hiatus hernia, whether small or large, is never on its own an indication for surgery, as invariably this report is dependent upon the technique and enthusiasm of the radiologist rather than on the conditions prevailing at the diaphragmatic hiatus. However, if the uncommon 'rolling' or para-oesophagal hernia (Figure 15) is present, then this usually requires surgical repair to avoid mechanical complications such as strangulation.

Patients who may best be treated for reflux surgically are:

- Those in whom medical treatment fails: some patients do not respond to medical treatment, even though they conscientiously comply with medical advice. If the patient's symptoms are severe enough, and he or she is fit enough, then surgery should be considered.
- Those who find it irksome to take medication continuously.

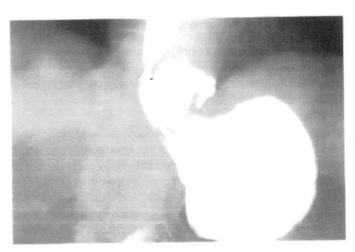

Figure 15
X-ray showing para-oesophageal (rolling) hernia.

- Those whose heartburn, pain, etc are controlled by medication but still have symptoms – regurgitation, cough, etc – from anacid reflux.
- Those who cannot be maintained on simple therapy: some patients may remain trouble-free only on a regimen that is too complicated or costly for long-term use and is incompatible with their lifestyle (eg, where bending or stooping is essential), or is just unacceptable to them.
- Those with troublesome concomitant abdominal disease: if a patient with reflux symptoms also has gallstones or a peptic ulcer requiring surgery, then an anti-reflux operation can be done at the same time.
- Some patients with complications: patients in whom reflux has caused ulceration or a stricture are most likely to need surgery, but these complications are far from absolute indications. Ulcers may heal surprisingly well without surgery, and strictures may melt away under the effects of proper medication combined with endoscopic dilatation. Results of dilatation of strictures are best when oesophagitis is also controlled.

Operations for reflux oesophagitis

Acid-reducing operations (e.g. vagotomy or partial gastrectomy) alone are unsatisfactory: excess acid is not the cause of reflux oesophagitis and acid secretion can be effectively inhibited by anti-secretory drugs.

Many procedures are used to reduce or to arrest gastro-oesophageal reflux. Each procedure has its enthusiasts and most are successful in the hands of their protagonists, but good results are achieved only in 70 to 80 per cent of patients when done by other surgeons. The most widely used and readily reproducible technique is fundo-plication (Nissen) in which a cuff of the gastric fundus is brought up round the lower oesophagus like an inkwell (see Figure 14). It is possible to do this operation by minimally invasive (laparoscopic) techniques. There was enthusiasm for a simple operation in which a silicone ring (the Angelchik prosthesis) is tied round the lower oesophagus sphincter to prevent reflux, but dysphagia often resulted and the prosthesis may migrate, so this is done less frequently now.

The belief that bile reflux is critically important in the causation of reflux oesophagitis has led to operations to divert bile, usually a Roux-en-Y anastomosis, particularly when access to the gastro-oesophageal region is technically difficult, but insufficient operations of this type have been carried out and their value is therefore difficult to assess.

Reflux in children

At birth the gastro-oesophageal barrier mechanism is poorly developed and all infants regurgitate easily. Sometimes this is severe and careful postural methods of control may be required. In most instances the barrier mechanism 'matures' and slowly becomes competent.

In a few infants easy regurgitation continues and this can damage health, both because of poor nutrition (when feeds are constantly regurgitated) or because of aspiration into the lungs causing pneumonia, pulmonary collapse, etc. Sometimes recurrent respiratory problems may be the main symptom of gastro-oesophageal reflux.

Investigation in infants is a special problem. Barium radiology may help, endoscopy may show oesophagitis, and it is possible to use intraluminal pH monitoring adapted to the infant's size.

Treatment also presents particular problems. Alginate compounds may be used, but with caution because of their relatively high sodium content. Anti-secretory drugs may also be used, but also with caution. Occasionally anti-reflux surgery is necessary.

Gastro-oesophageal reflux in pregnancy

Heartburn is extremely common in pregnancy, mainly because of hormonal effects on the gastro-oesophageal sphincter, accentuated by raised intra-abdominal pressure. It is unusual for this to give rise to significant oesophagitis unless there has been pre-existing reflux before pregnancy.

Because of pregnancy investigations are kept to a minimum, but if symptoms are severe it may be desirable to perform upper GI endoscopy.

In most instances simple antacids, perhaps combined with alginate compounds, are enough to control the symptoms until the end of pregnancy. If symptoms are severe consideration must be given to the use of anti-secretory drugs. These have been used only sparingly in pregnancy, so little evidence is available about possible adverse effects though none are specifically recognised. Both H_2-antagonists and proton pump inhibitors have been used, but should only be considered where symptoms are extreme and after careful discussion with obstetrician and patient.

The main complications of reflux are:

- Oesophageal ulcer

- Barrett's syndrome

- Benign oesophageal stricture (see page 48)

- Pulmonary complications including asthma (see page 13)

- Haemorrhage, which is uncommon (see page 13)

Oesophageal ulcer

A peptic ulcer, similar to a duodenal ulcer, can occur rarely in the squamous mucosa of the oesophagus, more often at the junction of squamous and columnar epithelium, or within the columnar epithelium. This may cause more persistent pain than the usual burning discomfort of reflux. Such ulcers should always be checked endoscopically to ensure their benign nature, but usually respond to medical treatment with anti-reflux medication, including anti-secretory drugs. Only occasionally is surgery required.

Barrett's syndrome

Norman Barrett of St Thomas's Hospital, London, described the circumstance when the tubular oesophagus, normally lined by squamous epithelium, is instead lined for part of its length by an abnormal, metaplastic columnar epithelium. It is not clear why this occurs and Barrett thought it was congenital. That is not so, and all these patients have reflux, often severely. They do not necessarily have symptoms. The condition is often discovered by chance, but the patient may have the usual symptoms of reflux.

The importance of the condition is that a benign ulcer may occur in the epithelium, sometimes leading to stricture. The metaplastic mucosa has a much higher likelihood than normal squamous epithelium of becoming malignant. Despite this knowledge, there is no agreement about the best management. Ulcers usually heal with medical therapy. Anti-reflux surgery, or potent anti-secretory drugs may produce some evidence of regenerating areas of squamous epithelium, but no major reversal of the abnormality. Some experts believe that regular endoscopic biopsies should be done to try to anticipate the development of malignancy, but this arduous life-time of endoscopy has not been demonstrated to be cost-effective.

Management points
- Most heartburn responds well to simple measures.
- Chest pain, even of 'anginal' type, may be from the oesophagus, and not the heart.
- Most gastro-oesophageal reflux responds well to medical treatment.
- Heartburn on its own usually arises from gastro-oesophageal reflux, but if there are additional symptoms (e.g. abdominal pain, dysphagia, vomiting, weight loss), or if simpler measures do not quickly bring relief, then investigation is necessary.
- Surgery is needed only in a few severe cases.
- The presence or absence of a hiatus hernia is not important, and the use of this term worries many patients unnecessarily.
- Before thinking of drugs and medicines, remember the importance of:
— reduction of excess weight
— avoidance of bending
— stopping smoking
— diminishing intake of fats, coffee, chocolate.

- Various therapeutic agents act by different mechanisms and, used logically in the right combination, they relieve most patients.
- Frequent antacids are the simplest form of treatment. Combined with an alginate reflux suppressant, they help most patients with mild disease.
- Acid-secretion blockers help most patients.
- Surgery should be reserved for those who have persistent symptoms despite full-scale medical treatment, or in whom such treatment cannot be sustained.

Dysphagia and Management of Carcinoma and Strictures

Background
Causes of dysphagia
Symptoms and diagnosis
Management

Difficulty in swallowing is a clear and recognizable symptom. Dysphagia always has an organic cause and should never be dismissed without investigation. Difficulty in initiating a swallow or the feeling of swallowed material 'sticking' or being delayed in its passage through the oesophagus should be differentiated from the following:

- Globus sensation: a feeling of a lump in the throat which does not interfere with swallowing but is not necessarily imaginary.
- Odynophagia: a sensation of pain or soreness as swallowed material (probably hot or alcoholic drink) passes down the gullet.
- Gastric fullness: this may be confused with a swallowing problem.

Although structural disorders (e.g. strictures, carcinomas, etc) are important causes of dysphagia, functional problems with disordered motility may be harder to diagnose yet equally deserving of treatment.

Causes of dysphagia

The main causes are:

•	Failure of the voluntary swallowing reflex
	Abnormalities of oesophageal motility
	Oesophagitis
•	Mechanical obstruction of the oesophagus

Failure of voluntary swallowing reflex

This can be divided into two groups: (1) voluntary (malingering) or psychogenic and (2) neurological.

Voluntary (malingering) or psychogenic
This condition is uncommon and, in young people, may be related to anorexia nervosa, while in the elderly it may reflect underlying anxiety and depression. It must be differentiated from a structural pharyngeal lesion. Even if the nature of the problem is unclear from the history, the radiologist may recognize that the patient makes inadequate attempts to initiate a swallow.

Neurological
This is seen in conditions such as motor neurone disease (in which the musculature of the tongue, pharynx and palate are

affected) and 'pseudo-bulbar palsy' (due to upper motor neurone lesions, usually associated with cerebrovascular disease). Myasthenia gravis and some myopathies may also affect the swallowing muscles. Careful history-taking will elicit whether the patient has had difficulty starting a swallow, if there has been any regurgitation into the nose, or if spill-over into the larynx has caused a cough. Examination of the tongue and palate may show wasting or diminished movement. Cinefilm or a video record of a barium swallow helps in analysis of the rapid movements which occur as the voluntary first stage of swallowing takes place.

Abnormalities of oesophageal motility

These are divided into: (1) crico-pharyngeal sphincter abnormalities, (2) loss of peristalsis, (3) spasm disorders, including achalasia.

Crico-pharyngeal sphincter abnormalities

The upper oesophageal sphincter is strong, but under voluntary control. If normal synchronous relaxation fails, it may cause obstruction to swallowing, sometimes with a radiologically visible 'crico-pharyngeal bar'. This in turn generates high pressures in the pharynx and may result in a pharyngeal diverticulum (Figure 16). If the resultant dysphagia is severe, surgical treatment may be needed, when it may be necessary not only to remove the diverticulum but to slit the sphincter (crico-pharyngeal myotomy). This condition is rare, and seen only in the elderly.

Loss of peristalsis

The normal progressive wave of peristalsis may be absent due either to a complete absence of contraction or to multiple contractions which occur in an uncoordinated manner ('spasm') (see Figure 11). Multiple contractions often occur in the elderly, while a complete absence of contraction is one manifestation of scleroderma. On its own it usually does not cause troublesome swallowing, but quite minor additional problems may lead

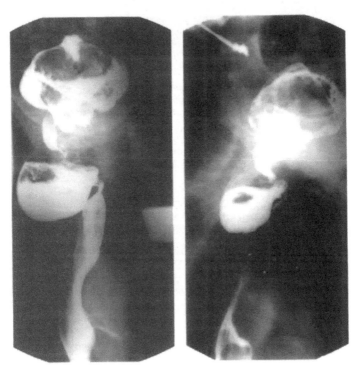

Figure 16
Barium swallow demonstrating a large pharyngeal diverticulum.

to trouble. For example, if the patient has to be confined to bed, the occurrence of oesophagitis or a small degree of extrinsic pressure may cause disproportionate dysphagia due to loss of peristaltic push.

Achalasia
In this uncommon condition (sometimes called cardio-spasm) the lower oesophageal sphincter does not relax and peristalsis is totally lost from the body of the oesophagus. The condition occurs gradually over many years and the classic picture is unmistakable, though some patients have been dismissed as psychoneurotic for years because progression is slow and they may describe their symptoms poorly (e.g. emphasizing regur-

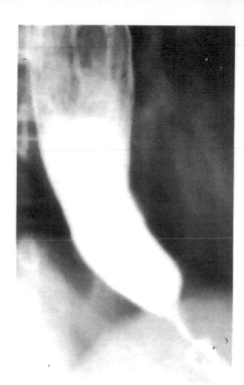

Figure 17
Barium swallow showing achalasia.

gitation and vomiting). Characteristically, there is a long history of progressive dysphagia for liquids and solids alike, together with regurgitation of undigested food. There may be episodes of spontaneous and severe chest pain. A barium swallow shows a widely dilated oesophagus with a tapered narrowing at the lower end (Figure 17). The diagnosis requires careful confirmation, certainly with endoscopy, to ensure nothing else is obstructing the lower end, and preferably pressure measurements (see Figure 11). Care is essential because treatment consists of deliberately damaging the gastro-oesophageal sphincter by forceful dilatation or surgical myotomy. This can be disastrous if the diagnosis is mistaken.

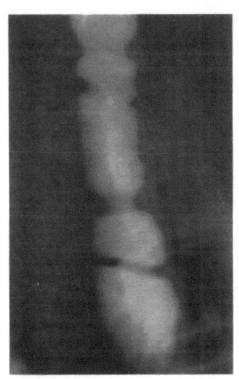

Figure 18
Barium swallow showing marked diffuse oesophageal spasm.

Oesophagitis

Oesophagitis may be due to oesophageal mucosal inflammation from any cause. In reflux oesophagitis, the inflammation sometimes interferes with normal motility so the peristalsis disappears and is replaced by abnormal spasm. This may cause swallowing difficulties, but dysphagia is usually mild, though it is worth looking for reflux as the cause of intermittent oesophageal spasm (Figure 18) as it is readily corrected. Severe dysphagia after a period of reflux oesophagitis usually means that a stricture has occurred (see page 48).

Infective oesophagitis

This is fairly uncommon. Rarely, viruses (e.g. herpes simplex) produce a transient oesophagitis with dysphagia, but the only infective oesophagitis seen with frequency is due to *Candida* (Monilia). This usually occurs in the elderly or debilitated, especially if they are on corticosteroids, immuno-suppressives or antibiotics and is frequent in patients with AIDS. This condition can cause severe dysphagia, but in the very ill patient it may not be recognized and deterioration ascribed simply to the serious primary illness. It is therefore important not to overlook infective oesophagitis for it can be readily treated and the patient's life saved. It may be seen on X-ray, but endoscopy shows it better as cheese-white plaques covering the whole oesophagus (see Figure 2). Smears or biopsies confirm the presence of fungal mycelia. It responds to nystatin, fluconazole or betaconazole.

Corrosive oesophagitis (see Figure 3)

This is due to inflammation caused by swallowing a caustic substance. It certainly causes dysphagia, but the reason is usually obvious. The material, often a household cleansing agent, may have been swallowed accidentally or with suicidal intention. A less obvious problem is that localized oesophagitis may be caused by a tablet that has stuck in the oesophageal mucosa and created a localized erosion. Many patients unwisely swallow tablets without water, especially at bedtime, and these stick in the gullet particularly of elderly patients whose peristalsis is disordered. Tetracycline and other antibiotics, potassium chloride and NSAIDs, (including the ubiquitious anti-thrombotic aspirin) particularly cause this problem. The characteristic syndrome is the sudden onset of central chest pain and severe dysphagia even for liquids. At endoscopy, a small round erosion (or less commonly a larger area of oesophagitis) is seen. The problem settles down spontaneously in a few days, but there is a risk that a stricture may result (see page 48).

Mechanical obstruction of the oesophagus

This may result from: (1) extrinsic pressure (2) foreign bodies (3) benign oesophageal strictures and rings or (4) carcinoma.

Extrinsic pressure

Various outside structures may press on the oesophagus and cause obstruction. For example:

- Enlarged left antrum

- Bronchial carcinoma

- Enlarged lymph nodes at the hilum of the lung

- Dilated aorta ('dysphagia aortica')

- Congenital abnormalities of the main thoracic arteries ('dysphagia lusoria') (see Figure 19)

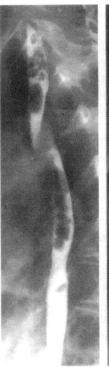
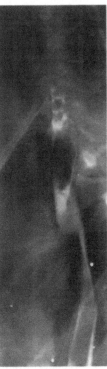

Figure 19
Barium swallow showing characteristic spiral deformity caused by aberrant subclavian artery.

Occasionally, extrinsic pressure may be present for some time without causing symptoms, and dysphagia results because oesophageal function starts to fail (e.g. old age). The diagnosis of an extrinsic cause is made by the associated symptoms and signs combined with expert radiology. All conditions are dealt with on their merits but, unless dysphagia is severe, may frequently be left untreated.

Foreign bodies
These should be considered if dysphagia occurs suddenly in a child or an unfit or demented elderly person. A foreign body does not usually impact in an adult oesophagus unless there is already some narrowing from either extrinsic pressure or perhaps an early stricture, although tablets are delayed for several minutes in their passage down the gullet.

Benign oesophageal strictures (Figures 20 and 22)
These are occasionally the result of swallowing corrosives, which is fortunately rare in Western Europe. In the UK almost all benign strictures are due to reflux oesophagitis which has been present for many years, producing slow and progressive damage; though strictures sometimes occur quickly in a patient who has been recumbent, especially with a nasogastric tube in place. Almost all benign reflux strictures occur in the elderly, the peak incidence being 65-75 years.

Webs and rings

Sideropenic dysphagia (Patterson-Brown-Kelly or Plummer-Vinson Syndrome)
In this rare condition there is a web in the upper oesophagus (Figure 21), usually associated with iron deficiency in older people (e.g. over 60 years of age). It must be differentiated from carcinoma, but is itself a pre-malignant condition so that a true carcinoma may follow months or years later.

Lower oesophageal rings (Schatzki-Kramer rings)
These can cause a characteristic syndrome of occasional

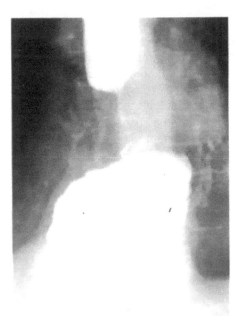

sudden dysphagia for a solid bolus, especially when the sufferer eats in public (e.g. a restaurant). The ring can be shown by careful radiology with good oesophageal distension, or by endoscopy. Bougie dilatation to 20 mm is usually effective treatment. All such strictures must be carefully inspected endoscopically, and biopsy and cytology specimens taken so that a carcinoma is not overlooked (Figure 22).

Carcinoma of the oesophagus

A squamous carcinoma may arise in the oesophagus or adenocarcinoma at the cardia, or in a segment of Barrett's metaplastic epithelium. Unfortunately the symptom of dysphagia usually occurs late because it does not take place until the growth has spread round, say, two-thirds of the lumen. By this point the growth is inevitably quite advanced (Figure 23). There is usually a sudden onset of dysphagia with impaction of a solid bolus, with rapid progress sometimes producing dysphagia for everything except small amounts of liquids. Radiology is not always reliable in diagnosis, particularly for carcinoma of the gastric fundus. Endoscopy is always essential (Figure 24), both to confirm a suspected carcinoma by biopsy, and if dysphagia is present without any clear radiological abnormality.

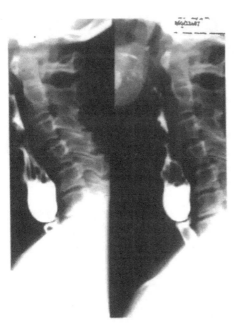

Figure 21
Barium swallow showing
an upper oesophageal
web.

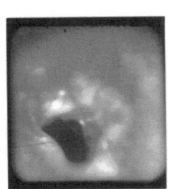

Figure 22
Endoscopic view of oesophageal
stricture with associated
oesophagitis.

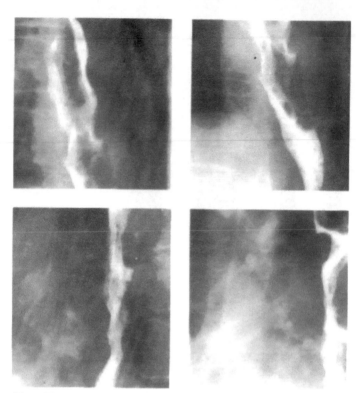

Figure 23
Barium swallow of an advanced oesophageal carcinoma showing irregular narrowing.

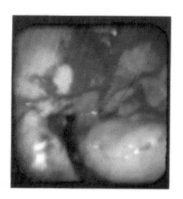

Figure 24
Endoscopic view of oesophageal carcinoma showing irregular narrowing.

Symptoms and diagnosis (Table 3)

It is often thought that the patient can accurately recognize the site at which an obstruction is occurring. This is not so, and many patients with obstruction at the lower end of the gullet may feel dysphagia in the throat. A careful analysis of the patient's symptoms (i.e. the rate of onset, speed of recovery and associated symptoms) is often an excellent guide to the precise nature of the abnormality, but confirmation by special investigation is always necessary.

Dysphagia must never be dismissed lightly. Unless it is confidently concluded that the patient's symptoms are imaginary, a barium swallow is desirable as the first step, together with a straight chest film. Cinefilms or video tapes can be helpful in analyzing barium swallows, especially when the voluntary swallowing mechanism is concerned or when a motility disorder is suspected.

Radiology alone is never sufficient. Endoscopy is essential to check any structural abnormality shown by X-ray and to take biopsy and cytology specimens from it, or to look for structural abnormalities not seen on the X-ray.

More complex tests (e.g. isotope scintiscan or pressure recordings) can help in occasional problem cases of motility disorders. Despite the availability of special tests a careful approach to diagnosis of symptoms is always helpful and the algorithm designed by Dr D.A.W. Edwards (Figure 25) indicates the critical questions that aid the process.

Table 3
Differential diagnosis.

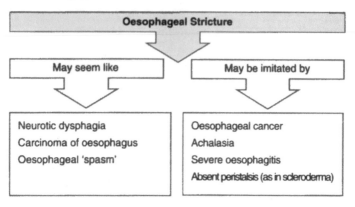

Oesophageal Stricture	
May seem like	**May be imitated by**
Neurotic dysphagia	Oesophageal cancer
Carcinoma of oesophagus	Achalasia
Oesophageal 'spasm'	Severe oesophagitis
	Absent peristalsis (as in scleroderma)

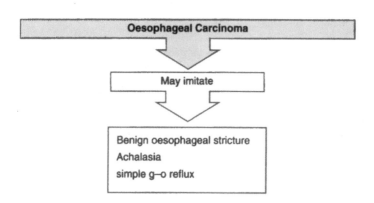

Oesophageal Carcinoma
May imitate
Benign oesophageal stricture
Achalasia
simple g–o reflux

The treatment of every cause of dysphagia cannot be discussed within the confines of this pocketbook, so attention is paid to the conservative management of benign strictures and approaches to carcinoma.

Benign oesophageal strictures

There are three choices available: (1) medical treatment alone (2) a combination of medical treatment with intermittent bougie dilatation or (3) surgery.

Medicine alone

Simply treating the reflux oesophagitis with medication and posture is sometimes enough to cause the stricture to resolve. Clearly, these strictures cannot be rigid, fibrous ones with peri-oesophagitis; they presumably have a major element of spasm and swelling owing to mucosal inflammation, which will disappear if treated adequately. Apart from administering medicines to reduce and neutralize reflux, it is important to stop drugs which may make things worse (e.g. NSAIDs or corticosteroids). Even if the stricture remains, healing the associated oesophagitis may produce a marked improvement in swallowing.

Figure 25
Algorithm for dysphagia.

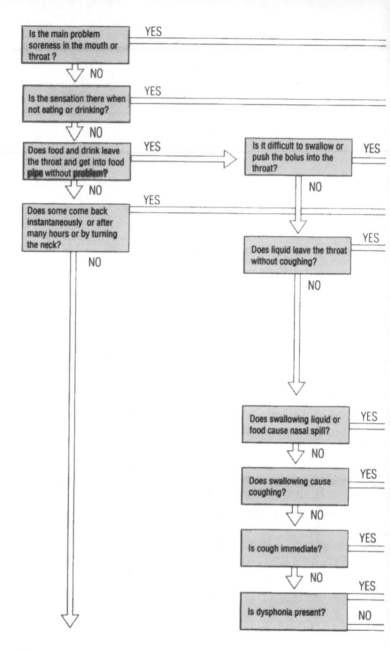

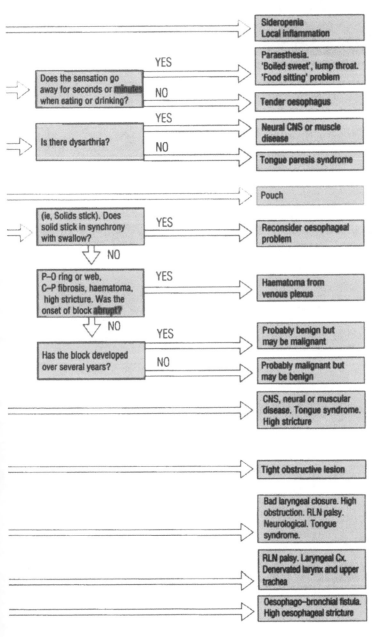

		Sideropenia Local inflammation
Does the sensation go away for seconds or minutes when eating or drinking?	YES	Paraesthesia. 'Boiled sweet', lump throat. 'Food sitting' problem
	NO	Tender oesophagus
Is there dysarthria?	YES	Neural CNS or muscle disease
	NO	Tongue paresis syndrome
		Pouch
(ie, Solids stick). Does solid stick in synchrony with swallow?	YES	Reconsider oesophageal problem
	NO	
P–O ring or web, C–P fibrosis, haematoma, high stricture. Was the onset of block abrupt?	YES	Haematoma from venous plexus
	NO	
Has the block developed over several years?	YES	Probably benign but may be malignant
	NO	Probably malignant but may be benign
		CNS, neural or muscular disease. Tongue syndrome. High stricture
		Tight obstructive lesion
		Bad laryngeal closure. High obstruction. RLN palsy. Neurological. Tongue syndrome.
		RLN palsy. Laryngeal Cx. Denervated larynx and upper trachea
		Oesophago–bronchial fistula. High oesophageal stricture

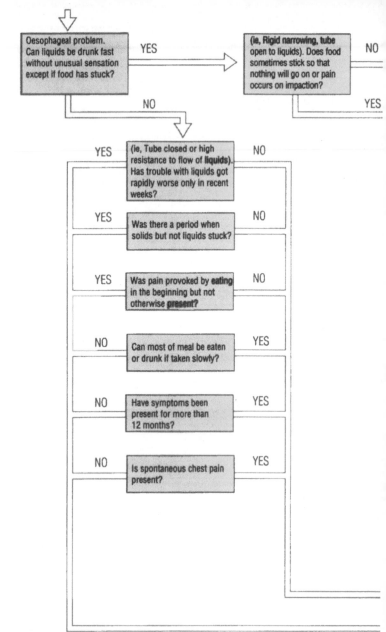

Oesophageal problem. Can liquids be drunk fast without unusual sensation except if food has stuck? — **YES** → (ie, Rigid narrowing, tube open to liquids). Does food sometimes stick so that nothing will go on or pain occurs on impaction? — **NO** / **YES**

NO ↓

(ie, Tube closed or high resistance to flow of liquids). Has trouble with liquids got rapidly worse only in recent weeks? — **YES** / **NO**

Was there a period when solids but not liquids stuck? — **YES** / **NO**

Was pain provoked by eating in the beginning but not otherwise present? — **YES** / **NO**

Can most of meal be eaten or drunk if taken slowly? — **NO** / **YES**

Have symptoms been present for more than 12 months? — **NO** / **YES**

Is spontaneous chest pain present? — **NO** / **YES**

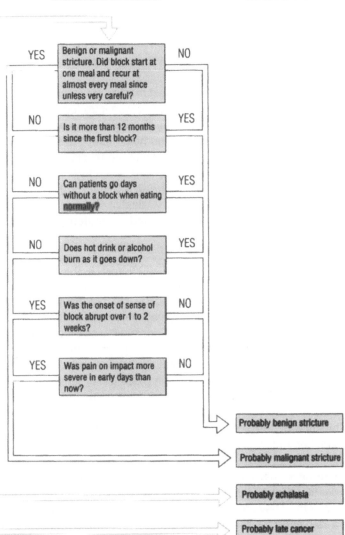

Does feeling that food is stuck come *after* eating and not during eating?

YES → Pseudodysphagia

NO → Achalasia

Benign or malignant stricture. Did block start at one meal and recur at almost every meal since unless very careful?   YES / NO

Is it more than 12 months since the first block?   NO / YES

Can patients go days without a block when eating normally?   NO / YES

Does hot drink or alcohol burn as it goes down?   NO / YES

Was the onset of sense of block abrupt over 1 to 2 weeks?   YES / NO

Was pain on impact more severe in early days than now?   YES / NO

Probably benign stricture

Probably malignant stricture

Probably achalasia

Probably late cancer

Bougienage

For most patients, good swallowing can be maintained by intermittent bougie dilatation, usually combined with medical anti-reflux treatment. As we have no method, at present for predicting the future behaviour of a stricture, it is best to start off with a few dilatations in any patient with a stricture. In the majority of patients, it will be possible to lengthen the intervals between dilatations quite quickly; many need only two or three initially, and subsequently less than one a year.

Dilatation The standard and safest method of dilatation is with a set of bougies passed over a guide-wire introduced through a fibreoptic endoscope. Radiological control may be used for added safety. The patient may go home later the same day, having only had some intravenous benzodiazepine and perhaps a little pethidine during the procedure. There are several good sets of dilators available (Figure 26): (1) wire-guided dilators (Eder-Puestow; Celestin; Savary: Key-Med Advanced Dilators), (2) balloons and (3) mercury-weighted bougies.

Wire-guided dilators These dilators use a guide-wire to achieve safety. The main hazard of stricture dilatation is that of oesophageal perforation caused by the bougie taking the wrong course. The guide-wire (with a flexible 'finger' at its end) is passed down through the stricture into the stomach, usually by being passed down the biopsy channel of a fibreoptic endoscope, but it can be done without endoscopy under radiological guidance. When the wire is in place (and the endoscope has been withdrawn) the bougies can be pushed over it to dilate the stricture, their position being ascertained by a combination of 'feel' and measurement, or by its progress being watched radiologically.

Balloons These are being used increasingly and are designed like those for angioplasty, so that they will not exceed a known diameter. They are passed under radiological control, filled with X-ray contrast material, or passed down the endoscopy

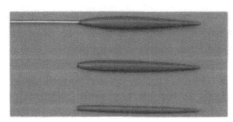

Figure 26
(a) KAD plastic dilators with diameters of 7 mm, 11 mm and 14 mm;

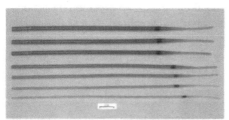

(b) Savary dilators;

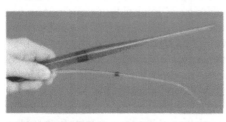

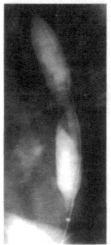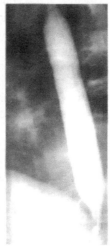

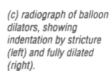

(c) radiograph of balloon dilators, showing indentation by stricture (left) and fully dilated (right).

channel and inflated with air under direct vision. They are breakable and more expensive than bougies; moreover, the relief of dysphagia by bougies usually lasts longer.

Weighted bougies Sir Arthur Hurst designed the well-known mercury-weighted dilator, which patients with strictures or achalasia can swallow daily to preserve their swallowing ability. However, in recent years they have been replaced by Maloney dilators, which are also mercury-weighted. The Maloney dilators are tapered at the tip and are becoming increasingly used in outpatient clinics, without sedation, passed by doctors or nurses or by patients in their own homes.

Surgery
Until the last 10 years, surgery was favoured for all but the unfit. However, the efficacy of intermittent bougienage has become increasingly clear and, as so many of the patients are elderly, the proportion treated by surgery these days is small, Surgery should be reserved for fit, young patients who have not done well on conservative treatment, or who find the treatment arduous. When surgery is undertaken, the stricture is not usually removed. Mostly it is sufficient to perform an anti-reflux operation, dilating the stricture at the time or later by bougies. If reflux is adequately prevented, oesophagitis resolves and the stricture opens up, or at least does not narrow, after dilatation.

Carcinoma of the oesophagus

Once the oesophageal carcinoma is fully diagnosed, three options are available: (1) surgery (2) radiotherapy and (3) palliation.

Surgery
Surgical extirpation of the growth offers the only real hope of a cure, although there are reports of long survival after radiotherapy. Unfortunately, the five-year survival in most series is well under 30 per cent, even when growths only suitable for radical surgery are included. If all growths are tackled, the

figures are dismal and some reports record a hospital mortality as high as 30 per cent. Resection of squamous oesophageal carcinoma has the highest mortality of any routine operation in the UK. Apart from the advanced state of growth at the time of diagnosis, the main reason for a poor outcome is the under-nourished state of the patient owing to his swallowing ability being so reduced. It is not within the scope of this book to suggest the best type of surgery; resection can be done in one, two or three stages, but it is always formidable surgery that requires not only high technical surgical skill, but also strong anaesthetic nursing and nutritional support and excellent post-operative care. These patients should only be operated on in units performing at least 25 cases a year. Careful selection of patients is important if this difficult and expensive surgery is to be used to its best advantage. If it is known that the growth is incurable, palliation by other methods should be seriously considered. However, it is equally important not to deny any chance of cure to a patient. Patients for surgical resection should nevertheless fulfil at least the following criteria:

- Histologically proven carcinoma
- No lung metastases on chest X-ray
- No liver metastases by ultrasound or CT scan
- Adequate respiratory reserve

Additional assessment of operability by MRI scanning, laparoscopy, and intraluminal ultrasound is being used increasingly. If the patient is aged over 70 years, or if the growth is more than 5 cm in length, then he or she should be considered with particular care, though neither of these criteria positively rules a patient out. If the carcinoma is of squamous type, however, the patient may do as well with radiotherapy.

Radiotherapy

Squamous carcinoma of the skin responds well to radiotherapy and it might be expected that squamous oesophageal carcinoma would also do well. Only a few centres have had good results but, for understandable reasons, they usually receive only those rejected for surgery. Meanwhile, it seems best to try radiotherapy for any patient with a carcinoma whose growth is extensive, or who is elderly, or unfit and therefore a risky candidate for major surgery. Additionally, surgery is not the correct course to take if there are known to be distant metastases because the life expectancy of these patients is so short that the discomfort and hazards resulting from major surgery cannot be justified. Radiotherapy maybe by a standard external beam technique, but intraluminal irradiation (brachytherapy) using the Selectron machine to insert radioactive pellets into a carefully sited tube within the oesophagus is quick and safe. It is not curative but can produce good palliation.

Palliation

Apart from the relief of pain by analgesia, palliation means overcoming the dysphagia so as to maintain the patient's nutrition and hydration until the spread of the growth finally results in death. The more normal the swallowing, the better the palliation. A particular problem for palliation is a tracheo-oesophageal fistula, which ensures early death if the connection between the gullet and airways is not sealed. Some of the techniques used during palliation are outlined below:

- Recurrent dilatation: simple dilatation, as for benign strictures, may be used recurrently to maintain the lumen. This can be helpful, but the frequency with which dilatation is required tends to increase, and this can become irksome to both patient and operator. There is also a risk of perforation on each occasion, so placement of a prosthetic tube is to be preferred, if at all possible.
- Endoscopic intubation: although for the past 25 years tubes have been introduced into oesophageal neoplasms through rigid endoscopes, current practice favours the use of fibreoptic endoscopes (see below).
- Disobliteration of the growth by laser, diathermy probe or alcohol injection (see below).

- Operative intubation: for many years, tubes of various materials (latterly plastic) were placed through the growths at laparotomy, being pulled down through a gastrostomy. Yet the morbidity and mortality of even this minor palliative procedure was high (up to 15 per cent mortality) because of the nutritional state of the patients. New methods of intubation using endoscopy have therefore been devised.
- Nasogastric feeding: if a prosthetic tube cannot be inserted for some technical reason, or if the growth is high and the tube could cause an unpleasant irritation in the throat, then hydration and nutrition may be maintained by the introduction of a soft polythene feeding tube 1 mm in diameter. This is done using a guide-wire under X-ray control, or by towing it into place with an endoscope. Liquid feed can be given by a continuous drip using gravity of a pump.
- Gastrostomy: this used to be dismissed as an undesirable technique, but modern percutaneous endoscopic gastrostomy (PEG) gives good opportunities for nutritional support, though swallowing remains severly limited.

Endoscopic intubation

The principle behind this technique is that the tube be advanced into position over a guide to avoid perforation. This guide may be a bougie, a steel wire, or the endoscope itself. It is essential to use intubation for a tracheo-oesophageal fistula so as to block off the abnormal communication.

Professor Michael Atkinson designed the Nottingham introducer (Figures 27 and 28), which grips the prosthetic tube from within. The silastic Atkinson or plastic Wilson-Cook tube is normally used, both of which are designed to avoid displacement either upwards or downwards, once inserted. There are also self-expanding metal-mesh stents, which are simpler to introduce but much more expensive.

The procedure may be performed with general anaesthesia, or using sedation with a benzodiazepine and pethidine (especially if the patient is very weak, or has respiratory disease).

The patient is not allowed to drink immediately, hydration being maintained by intravenous fluid. After 6-24 hours a radiological examination is performed to check the position of the tube and

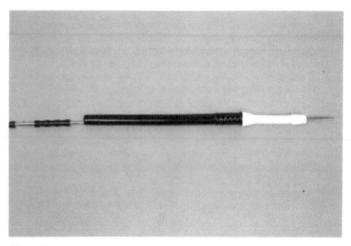

Figure 27
White silastic tube mounted on a Nottingham introducer for insertion into an oesophageal carcinoma.

to search for any evidence of perforation. If all is well, then clear fluids are permitted and the patient may gradually progress to a semi-solid diet, as long as he or she can chew well; alternatively, a liquidized diet should be introduced. To avoid blockages, meals should also be accompanied and followed by copious fizzy drinks.

Complications Perforation occurs in up to 10 per cent of introductions, usually because the growth has split during dilatation. This does not mean a disaster, provided it is recognized. The tube may still be introduced to seal the hole, but antibiotics must be given until radio-opaque fluid can be seen not to leak. Food may also impact in the tubes, which are usually only 11-12 mm in diameter. Effervescent drinks and swallowing diluted hydrogen peroxide may clear them. If not, the block must be dug or rammed out with an endoscope. Additionally, displacement may occur. Should an upwards displacement occur, this would necessitate removal of the tube and insertion of a new one. Distal displacement into the stomach is a nuisance, but best left alone unless there are symptoms; in which case, a new tube

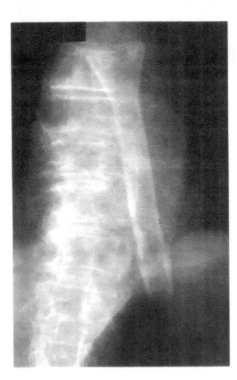

Figure 28
X–ray showing Atkinson
tube in situ.

should be inserted. Sometimes the old tube may be removed through the dilated growth, but this is a difficult procedure.

Metal-mesh stents (Figure 29) These come with a special introducer and are put in place under radiological control; they open to full diameter spontaneously or by inflation with a balloon. They are undoubtedly useful in certain special circumstances (e.g. high tumours where a plastic tube would be intolerable; nevertheless, cost effectiveness for all circumstances has not been proved.

Survival Although only intended for palliation of terminal disease, many patients survive months, or occasionally a year or two, with such tubes in place.

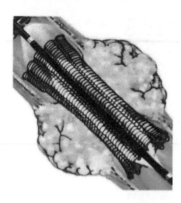

Figure 29
Metal-mesh balloon shown
diagrammatically. (By courtesy of
Boston Scientific Ltd.)

Disobliteration of the growth Nodules of tumour encroaching
on and narrowing the lumen can be burned away using a laser
beam directed through an endoscope under direct vision. Skill
is needed to obtain a good result, but in practised hands results
are good and perforation uncommon. Several sessions are
needed, and this can be exhausting both for patient and operator.

A similar effect can be obtained using a special probe heated
by diathermy current. This is less expensive because the high
capital cost of the laser source is avoided. It is not certain
whether it is effective as laser therapy.

Even cheaper and simpler is to slough the growth by multiple
small injections of absolute alcohol. Again, several sessions
are needed, and its efficacy compared with other palliative
techniques is not fully assessed.

Management points

- Never brush off a complaint of dysphagia. It always needs investigation. Disorders of function often cause dysphagia, but if it is constant and progressive, a structural abnormality such as stricture or carcinoma is likely.
- Barium studies alone may mislead; every patient with dysphagia needs an endoscopy as well.
- Be sure that a stricture is benign; histology and cytology are essential.
- Bougie dilatation in practised hands is safe and comfortable. The interval between dilatation usually lengthens out acceptably.
- Carcinoma of the oesophagus needs thoughtful assessment. Radical surgery is reserved for the potentially curable. For the remainder an increasing number of palliative procedures are available.

Appendix: Drugs and Doses

Drug and action	Genetic name and dosage	
Prokinetics (strengthen sphincter, speed gastic emptying)	Metoclopramide 10 mg Domperidone 10–20 mg Cisapride 5–10 mg	20–30 min before food and at bedtime
Alginate– antacid preparations (mechanically diminish reflux)	2 tablets or 100 ml suspension	After meals and at bedtime
Antacids (neutralize acid)	Preferably in tablet form	Suck one every 1–2 hours
Histamine–H_2-antagonists (reduce volume and acidity of gastric contents)	Ranitidine 300 mg Famotidine 40 mg Cimetidine 400 mg	At bedtime or twice daily Four times daily
Proton Pump Inhibitor (marked or complete reduction of acid secretion)	Omeprazole Lansoprazole	20–40 mg with breakfast 30 mg with breakfast

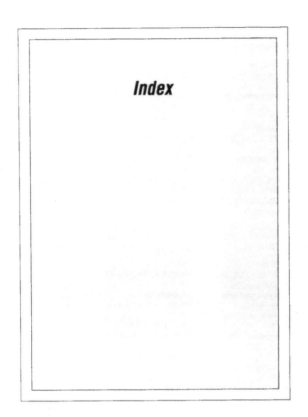

Index

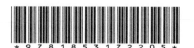

T - #0383 - 101024 - C80 - 191/121/5 - PB - 9781853172205 - Gloss Lamination